Exercising Kingdom Dominion in Dance

Professor Marilyn T. Deveaux, PhD.

TATE PUBLISHING, LLC

Dedication

The year 1994 was a season of bittersweet, unspeakable joy for me. My father died in March of that year, and instead of walking me through the valley of grief, my heavenly Father chose to release in me a floodgate of artistic creativity, in the form of poetry, songs, choreographies, plays and eventually my first major theatrical dance production. Thus, I dedicate this book to:

My Heavenly Father who continues to mold me into a vessel that is fit to carry and release His treasured gifts to the world;

John D. Deveaux, my earthly father, now asleep, whose passion for the performing arts continues to influence and inspire me; and

Elzena Deveaux, my mother, also asleep, who supported me constantly with encouragement through this and all my projects until her passing in September 2005.

Acknowledgements

During the period of the writing of this book, I was privileged to attend the retirement ceremony of the first Man of God to influence my life. It was a pleasure to sit again in the pews where I had grown up and sing familiar songs. In an age where materialism and immorality plague many Christian leaders, it was particularly rewarding to sit in that service and reminisce over the life and ministry of a man who served God with noted humility, simplicity, gentleness and freedom from the slightest hint of a scandal.

My heartfelt gratitude is extended to Rev. Dr. Garnet King, for teaching me by example how to serve God in like manner. Your favorite exhortation, "Doing increases the power of doing"–is a daily boost in times of frustration and weariness. Special thanks also to Dr. King's successor, Rev. Dr. Stephen E. Thompson and the Transfiguration Baptist Church fellowship, for your continued support to me and the VIRTUE Dance Academy vision.

To Dr. Myles Munroe, thank you; for under your leadership I learned the value of my unique potential, purpose, vision, leadership capacity and kingdom call.

To Bishop Neil C. Ellis, I am grateful to you for showing me the depth of the scripture that propels me to "Arise, shine, for (my) light has come."

To Pastor Rick Dean, thank you for your continued shepherding and practical teaching of how to apply kingdom principles in daily living. Special thanks also to "The Family" at Family Of Faith Ministries International, especially Sis. Gaye Dean.

To Dr. Blake Carlson, a true mentor, I owe you a depth of gratitude for your timely influence in my life to push me into a higher level of achievement, creativity and focus; which among other things resulted in the decision to write and complete this first manuscript.

To the parents of students of VIRTUE Dance Academy whose continued patronage has kept the doors of VIRTUE opened since 1997; your dancing darlings are like "permanent fixtures" in the studios of VIRTUE. Special thanks to Theresa Mortimer, Joy Simmons, Barbara Taylor, Lolitta Rolle, Lorieann Butler, Verona Pratt, Vanria Edwards, Orient Edgecombe, Shasta Major, Saskia Black and Miriam Curling.

To Tia Johnson, my "right-hand" assistant, you are a perpetual blessing to me both in the execution of your own dance call and your service to this great vision.

To my adult students and assistants–Shanrese Bain, Dominique Bain, Germaine Demeritte and Katurah Johnson–thank you for being willing and available to function as students and teachers in the development of our curriculum and resources.

To my former students who have moved on to either begin your own–or assist in the building of another's–dance vision. Thanks to you all–Mervin Smith, Lucille Bassett, Kendra Arnette, Nicole Bowe, Candy Curtis and Samantha Cox–for your commitment during your season with VIRTUE.

To Natalie Allen - VIRTUE's first international Degree candidate who resides in Baker Hill, Montserrat - thanks for your input in encouraging me to complete this book and not to procrastinate, but *"to move with the cloud on this one."* Special thanks also to the exciting group of Christian dance leaders from around the world who are currently–or were previously–enrolled in our VSC and/or Degree certification programs; especially Tamara Finlayson-Fuller (Jamaica), April Bell (USA), Tamika Sudler (USA), Lorraine Coote (Jamaica), Virgen Morales (USA), Marcia Brunson (USA), Vickie Caldwell (USA), Sue Hartley (Australia) and Kishawn Banks (USA).

To my best friends whom I have known for most of my life, I thank you all - Yvette Cooper, Elsa Roker, Deta Miller, Anthony & Debbie Lopez - for inspiring, encouraging, "interceding-on-behalf-of" and (when necessary) rebuking me. Special thanks also to Dandria Scott, Elga Miller and Joan Knowles.

To the members of my immediate family, thanks for your love and support–Dorothy, Leroy, Robert & Jermaine. Special thanks also to Kelly Hamilton and Joycelyn Deveaux.

To those vendors–Stephanie Saunders and Michael Cartwright–whose favour has helped to keep the business of VIRTUE open - especially during the rocky periods - I pray God's blessings over you and your establishments.

To the Tate Publishing Team–especially Ryan, Jesika, Dave, Julie, Lindsay and Rita - thank you for believing in this project and for your excellent contributions in bringing it to fruition.

Finally, I extend my sincerest thanks to a certain individual whose search for the information contained in this book was the impetus for God's assigning me this writing task to begin with. To you, dear reader, I offer thanks for placing demands on God so that He would place demands on me to complete this first volume.

Contents

Chapter 1:

Enlarging Your Territory - An Overview

There is much talk nowadays about the next move of God in The Church. Some say it is the **prophetic season**, the **apostolic dispensation**, and even more say that it is the **age of the layman**. While there are merits to the postulations of these and other schools of thought, one thing must be remembered about the God whom we serve. HE CHANGES NOT. He is the same yesterday, today and forever.

When He walked the earth over 2000 years ago in the person of Jesus the Christ, He accomplished three main earthly goals:

> • *To set the captives free* through His life,
>
> • *To lead captivity captive* through His death, and
>
> • *To give gifts to men* through His resurrection.

The purpose of these gifts is contained in His final directive to His followers, to "go into all the world and make disciples." This "Great Commission" is or should be the blueprint, master plan, ultimate goal of every believer in these last days.

Much of the emphasis in the area of Christian Dance, since its restoration a few decades ago, has been placed on the priestly role such as liturgical or church ministry. Thus much of the literature, resources, and workshops have consistently produced little more than Bible studies for Christian dancers. There is no comprehensive focus on dance as an art form, plus its relation to culture, evangelism, industry, academia and research. All of these aspects of dance should be examined from the Christian perspective of The Great Commission.

Nevertheless, a great debt of gratitude is owed to those dance ministers and authors who have participated in the restoration, expansion, and education in this field. They have laid down a strong foundation to be built upon by emerging ministers such as myself during this evangelistic move of God in the end-times. As their students and protégés everywhere in The Body of Christ, we say "Thank you for so blessing us that we too might be a blessing."

To those of you who are just entering the ministry of dance, and are minimally aware of the struggle for restoration, acceptance and order that was the experience of our pioneers, then please do the right thing and read the works of these authors, seminar presenters, etc. at your local Christian bookstore, over the internet or abroad.

Now, *all formalities done,* Kingdom Dancer, I urge you to set aside some free time this month to go through this whole text plus the e-Seminar. It is not only the reading of the text that will bring about transformation in your life but also your full participation in the coursework–please see the Dominion Dancer e-Seminar Series Resources at the end of this book, and also visit our website at www.DominionDancer.com. My goal is to aid in the process of you experiencing your enlarged territory in dance. To get started, you will need a short history lesson, therefore, please proceed to look at the *Historical Backdrop and Contemporary Issues in Christian Dance.*

Chapter 2
Historical Backdrop & Contemporary Issues

The field of DANCE is a multifaceted industry that has exhibited tremendous growth during the last century and shows strong signs of staying on this continuum. Progressing from its technical roots in the court of the fifteenth century French King, its structure and language is well developed today in both the classical ballet tradition and the less rigid modern forms.

Beyond the entertaining, aesthetic, and inspirational influences of theatrical dancing, this art form offers nation-building value. Through formalized and continuing education, a career path in dance in the secular world could be charted from toddler to retirement, progressing from kinder-dance classes, through grade school, college, professional dancing, summer intensives and teaching.

Professional dance companies have always relied on funding from private and government sources, but the industry's economic growth in the 20th century could be attributed to revenues earned from such services and products as the operation of dance schools, major performances, summer programs, competitions, conventions, copyrights of original techniques and presentations, multi-media merchandise and dancewear manufacturing and sales.

In the area of Christian dance, the potential for growth is also phenomenal. The ministry of dance has its roots in Jewish rather than Christian traditions, but has nevertheless been restored to a place of recognition in the Body of Christ over the last three decades. The focus, however, has been mostly on liturgy, or liturgical dancing within the "four-walls" of the Church building. But if we really want to reach the world with the Gospel through dance, and if we are truly serious about funding the end-time harvest, then our thinking must be transformed from this *"four-walls-only" approach.*

Chapter 3
Ministry & Industry Considerations

There exists a hindrance in the *"four-walls-only"* narrow style of church dancing, which is described in such limiting terms as *"liturgical,"* *"praise,"* *"interpretive."* In some churches today, Christian dance is still relegated to little more than hand waving, rocking and kneeling in accompaniment to praise music, or contractions and emotional interpretation of popular gospel music. Thus, the appreciation of Christian dance begins and ends in the four walls of the Church, losing the artistic appeal that draws the general public to secular dance theatre.

Whenever I tell someone that I run a Christian dance school, they look at me as if to say, *"Yes and . . . what is your day job?"* The assumption is that this is not a serious, viable profession, but a *"mere ministry"* or side job. **Nevertheless, I**

believe that the ministry of movement is on the brink of a mighty move of God, pun intended. Dance is poised to become a vibrant evangelistic and commercial instrument for the training of dance ministers and the funding of local and global dance missions.

Just like the rise of the gospel music recording industry, so too will Christian dance theatre be elevated to industry standards in communities worldwide. And there is a strategic reason for this; for the Gospel according to Dance will go where the spoken Gospel cannot. Let me explain . . .

As the Church embarks on major worldwide missions, so too is secular society engaging in major "evangelistic" campaigns. Although many sectors and political groups are vying for attention to their individual agendas, they are all unified in one issue, which is that of their father the devil - *to silence the voice and influence of the Church in modern society.* The Word of God, whether uttered in sermons, prayers, scripture readings, or even in song, is being increasingly challenged as offensive and out-dated by secular society. (Nevertheless, who can challenge the testimony of a man whose life has visibly changed from an encounter with Christ?)

Among Jesus' last words when he walked the earth were those of the **Great Commission**, admonishing His servants to go into *all the world* and preach the gospel. Some preachers state that "world" here is not merely territorial, but refers to *"every sphere"* of society, *or "every man's world."* Thus, we see living testimonies of God's Word at work in converts from every field: Athletes can be heard in televised interviews glorifying God for their victories, artists attributing their works to Jesus in the music industry, and business people thanking God for giving them witty inventions that propel them to the top of their industry.

The area of visual and performing arts is another such "world," poised to become a major contributor to   ushering in the next wave of harvest. In particular, Christian dance can be a very effective evangelistic tool in this 21st century; however, the propensity for mediocrity, as demonstrated over the last two decades, must be eliminated. The Church must produce dancers who are not only anointed for "in-church" ministry but also dancers **whose excellence in technique and artistry exceeds - rather than equals - that of secular dance professionals in theatre settings**.

Throughout the 2000 years of church history, we see men and women of God establishing and creating whole new professions by God's creative power. It was Christians who established the nursing profession and hospitals for public healthcare, education for the masses, modern democratic political governance and superb fine arts - for e.g. Shakespeare in literature, Michelangelo in painting. Do you know that the most significant contributor in the fine art of music was a Christian composer? He is hailed as the Father of modern music whose genius is unsurpassed. It is said that he left no musical form as he found it and that he said the last word on everything he created. And guess what? According to one critic, he attributed every note he composed to Jesus Christ. **Will it be you who establish or greatly expand the boundaries of dance in general, just like Johann Sebastian Bach did for music during his lifetime?**

Chapter 4
Discovering Your Specific Domain

There is a popular Bahamian Christian song performed by the group "Christian Massive" called *"Know Your Role."* I like the chant at the end where the lead says, "I hope you know yours," and the back-ups echo "I hope you know yours too." It is a reminder that we must all find and continually walk in our calling, whatever it may be, and challenge each other to do so as well.

Christians tend to be too general when describing their ministry call, mission, or mission statement. We use phrases such as: "I am called to win the lost at any cost . . . to win the world for Jesus . . . to go into all the world and preach the gospel."

My mental response each time I hear that is, "That is not *your* mission, that's *my* mission, and our Kenyan *sister's* mission, and our Russian *brother's* mission." **It is really the mission of every born again believer; see Acts 1:8.**

But every born again believer is not called to win the lost in Alberta, Canada, or convert the Jamaican citizens for Jesus, or preach the gospel in Paris, France. So here is where specificity of mission applies.

Most of us are familiar with the *"Kingdom Teaching" that Jesus is The King of Kings, and that we are the kings that He is "King of."* Yes, the separate leadership roles in the Old Testament, namely, prophet, priest and king, are combined in each believer. So, I ask you, what is a king without a kingdom? Have you ever wondered what you are "king of"? Or, what is your domain/territory?

Dr. Turnel Nelson of Trinidad has an interesting interpretation of John 14: 1-4, that resonated deep in my spirit when I first heard it, *although not a popular interpretation.* Let us examine the scripture text first:

> *"Let not your heart be troubled; you believe in God, believe also in Me. In My Father's house are many mansions; if it were not so, I would have told you. I go to prepare a place for you.*

> *And if I go and prepare a place for you, I will come again and receive you to Myself; that where I am, there you may be also. And where I go you know, and the way you know."*

Dr. Nelson postulates that the **"mansions" Jesus** refers to are not literal edifices in the heavens, but are **domains**, or **offices**, to which every believer is assigned. In other words, we each hold a **recognizable office** in the Kingdom of God, a **special assignment** that only a specific individual can perform, that is **our place of authority and dominion in the earth**.

One of the buzz-words in the corporate world in the 1990s was **"core competency."** Businesses seeking high profitability were encouraged to stick to activities that were within their core competencies and conversely, to avoid others that were outside their core competencies. The principle is the same for individuals; **find your assigned office, domain, and specialized skill/service and exclusively cultivate it to Olympian perfection.**

Some Christian teachers are now describing it as **"your high calling."** The concept is explained in this example: If you are called to be a plumber and have all the skills, genius and passion to prove so - then by choosing to become a doctor instead you will have walked beneath your calling, and chosen a "lower" one.

It is very important that you discover your unique role, domain, office, core competency, or high calling in general, and particularly in the multifaceted area of Christian Dance.

To determine your unique office in Christian Dance, we will borrow from the Journalism field the **5W-1H questions** which reporters use to write interesting news stories; namely, who, what, where, when, why and how. These same questions are useful in helping you discover your dance ministry call in terms of **your assigned relationships, gifts, territory, time, purpose, and resources**. Below is an outline of these questions and answers. We will elaborate on the answers in the remaining chapters of this book.

WHO: To whom are you called? The answer to this question lies in the three main LAYERS of ministry: that is ministry unto (a) God alone, (b) the Church, (c) unbelievers.

WHAT: Exactly what are you called to do? The

"what" is determined by your unique gift, talent, ability, or potential.

WHERE: *Where is the locale of your call?* Territories include the church setting, theatre stages, public parks, your country, other countries, and the internet.

WHEN: *How much time can you commit to this call?* Dance requires much preparation in terms of consecration, rehearsal, training, and fellowship with team members.

WHY: *What is your purpose?* To which "work(s) of the ministry" and/or "five-fold leadership" roles *in dance* are you called?

HOW: *How will you administer your call?* You will need: (a) resource tools such as dance classes, rehearsals, workshops, books, videos, seminars and degree certification; (b) advancement skills such as technique, artistry, ministry and professional development; and (c) weapons such as the whole armor of God and a strong relationship with Him.

We will start with the "why" in the next chapter.

Chapter 5
The Order Of Ministry & Assignment

Jesus established a new order of ministry service when He introduced His Kingdom to the earth. I call it the *"trilogy of ministry"* because it involves three mandatory areas of assignment for every believer. We see this trilogy exemplified in His training of the disciples and later His commissioning of them.

First he called the disciples to Himself for training (Matthew 4:19), then He sent them on mission to their Jewish brethren (Matthew 10:5), and then He sent them to the gentiles, (Luke 10:1). Jesus repeated this ministry trilogy when informing the disciples of their new assignments to be executed after His ascension. Again, He first called them to wait in the upper room for empowerment by the Holy Ghost baptism (Acts 1:4), then sent them on the Great Commission, again firstly to their Jewish brethren (Acts 1:8a), and finally to the utmost parts of the world (Acts 1:8b).

Similarly, Christian dance (just like all other fields) follows this same ministry order, having three main assignments as per:

(1) **Audiences** - God, believers and non-believers;

(2) **Influences** - spiritual, emotional and sensual;

(3) **Ministry types** - private, liturgical and theatrical; and

(4) **Settings** - home, church building, community.

Private dancing unto God is a solo ministry before a solo audience of Jesus the King of Kings and can be done in the privacy of your own home or at your studio, church, or wherever you can spend this quality solitary time. The "audience" in this setting is concerned with the heart and passion of your presentation to Him. The aim is to worship and please the King, thus the influence and appeal are purely spiritual.

Liturgical dancing has its place in the "four-walls" boundary of the church, or any setting outside the church building where the gathering is likely to be at least 70% Christian. The aim is to execute priestly functions of invoking an atmosphere of praise and worship and testimony of God's gracious acts. The dancer is both familiar and comfortable with the audience in this setting - *as were the disciples on their first mission to the Jews.* The influence and appeal then is equally spiritual and emotional, and minimally sensual.

Theatrical Dance, for the most part, is presented outside the church walls, before non-believers in a cultural, theatrical or evangelistic setting. The aim is to present the gospel in an artistic way - i.e. not so much "churchy," but in the way of "salt" and "light" (Matthew 5:13-16). The audience in this type setting is not so forgiving of improper technique and minimized artistry, as they are already exposed to higher performance quality from the secular dance world. This type ministry employs both spiritual and emotional influences but with a larger component of entertaining, aesthetic tools such as advanced choreography design and technique that would be more visually attractive to a secular audience.

Please note that no part of the trilogy of ministry is optional. We are all called to minister first unto God, next to the brethren, and then to the world. Nevertheless two things must be remembered. Firstly, we do still have a specific call or area of dominion that may not be in all three of these realms, but just one. We will discuss this further in the next chapter. Secondly, although all three assignments are of equal importance, the third one must now take precedence in these last days. Why?

Evangelism is paramount for all sectors of the Body of Christ today. Remember that we have an eternity to look forward to worshipping God among the brethren, but only limited time–*for our days are like grass (Psalm 103:15)*–to win sinners for Christ; thus this should be the essential portion of our tri-part ministry assignment. **The first two are the means of equipping us for the real "work of the ministry"** particularly to sinners, which we will discuss in the next chapter.

As much as we desire and pray for God's presence to show up in our worship services, that is NOT God's ultimate plan for us on earth in this dispensation. Is it mentioned anywhere in the scriptures that angels rejoice over the visitation of the glory of God in our midst? No, my friend, **the heavenly party occurs when just one sinner is converted** (Luke 15:7).

However, that is not to diminish the desire and need for God's glory in our gatherings, **but we must maintain a balanced understanding that His presence must always be sought so that we will be enabled and empowered to carry out the Great Commission.** As it was in the beginning (i.e. on the day of Pentecost when 3000 souls were added to the Church) so let it be in these end times, that when we leave our glorious gatherings we will so impact the world that thousands of new converts will be birthed, not daily, but hourly.

The father desires new disciples. I remember the words of a popular gospel song in the eighties:

"My house is filled but my fields are empty.
Who will go and work for me today?
Oh, it seems like my children want to stay
around my table,
And just a few want to work in my field.
A faithful few want to work in my field."

Kingdom dancer, there is a ripe harvest out there (Luke 10:2) and all of our work will come to naught if we do not first equip ourselves in communion with God and the saints so that we can ultimately participate in the gathering-in of this end-time harvest.

Chapter 6

The Purpose Of Christian Dance–two Tiers

When we look at the Body of Christ at large, it is understood that every saint is a priest, king, and minister and is commissioned to disciple the people in his or her immediate world (i.e. co-workers, family members, friends and strangers). We all received our "great commissioning." But when it comes to one's specific calling, **two tiers of ministry** emerge, namely, the *"work of the ministry"* and *"five-fold ministry,"* which I will refer to as *"labour"* and *"leadership" ministries*, respectively.

The first tier, "work of the ministry," involves the "labour" of every single believer. We all have individual assignments that vary in terms of relationships (e.g. to kids or battered people), territory (as pertaining to a certain country, e.g. India), and gifts (as with the operation of our vocational or artistic gifts, e.g. nursing or singing).

The second tier, "five-fold ministry," involves believers that are specially endowed with such leadership gifts as apostleship, prophecy, evangelism, pastoral and teaching. Five-fold "leadership" ministers are charged with equipping the "labouring" saints, resulting in the edification of the Body of Christ at large. In other words **when five-fold ministers equip the saints, who then "work their ministry," corporate advancement of God's Kingdom is eminent.**

These same two tiers of service are replicated in the particular ministry area of dance. The first tier involves *six main labouring categories, or "works of the dance ministry," namely:*

- **In-church ministry, including praise/ worship, presentational, and prophetic dancing, along with mime and banner/ flag pageantry.**

- **Special events, theatrical and evangelistic missions outside the church setting.**

- **Industries such as dance school operation, teaching profession, consultancy and costume manufacturing and sales.**

- **Higher education, such as degree and certification programs.**

- **Continuing education, such as workshops, seminars and conventions.**

- **Multimedia Resources, such as books, instructional manuals, tapes, videos, websites, networks, etc.**

Likewise, second-tier dance ministers have leadership functions just like their equivalent five-fold ministers of the corporate Body of Christ as per Ephesians 4:7-16 as follows:

1. Apostles - Founders of dance ministries and networks, conference hosts, mentors of dance leaders.

2. Prophets - Praise & Worship, spontaneous, prophetic and presentational ministers in dance, mime, sign and pageantry (i.e. banners and flags).

3. Evangelists - Consultants, solo ministry artists, guest choreographers, seminar speakers.

4. Pastors - Dance leaders.

5. Teachers - Technique/choreography teachers, dance authors, professors and theologians.

Again, **the two purposes in the context of dance are that the five-fold leadership ministers equip all "labouring" dancers with skills and tools for the latter to perform their individual "work of the ministry"(see categories above), thus resulting in the edification, inspiration and encouragement of the Body of Christ at large.**

The key to effectiveness is for the dance leader to identify his/her five-fold dance ministry call(s) and to adapt his/her leadership style to that of the equivalent general Body of Christ role. In other words, if you're a guest choreographer, or consultant, then study and pattern your leadership style after the role of the evangelist; if you are just a dance leader, then shepherd your dance members as does a pastor with his flock.

Can you identify your area(s) of calling from the above groupings?

Chapter 7:

Gifts & Potential

The "what" question of determining your dance call is answered by what emerges in your life as your unique gift, talent, ability, or potential. Some dancers are very **technically proficient**, having trained for numerous years before and after their conversion. Some may not have had the opportunity to be trained, but they possess the ability or **potential to learn dances quickly**, and can thus advance quickly if given the opportunity to get training. Others may have no ability or interest in dance technique, but **can certainly execute - or even choreograph** - beautiful and anointed presentations.

Some dancers are **neither technically, or choreographically capable**. They simply cannot remember dance steps; but Oh how they can dance spontaneously, or prophetically. There are others also who can only sway from side to side, but give them a **flag, or a banner**, and you can expect to see the Glory of God rain down on their ministry offering.

Some may be more suited to mime, warfare, private worship, and theatre. Some may not be dancers at all but sense a strong affiliation with this fine arts ministry and can **contribute through such gifts as intercession, prophecy, teaching, administration and design/manufacturing of garments, costumes, banners and flags.**

For both efficiency and effectiveness of the dance ministry team, please be aware of these vital keys:

1) Stay in your individual area of domain and out of the others. If you are spontaneous, for instance, stay out of the choreographies and exhaust all your energy on your spontaneous presentations. If mime is your thing, then leave the flags to those of the pageantry team and perfect your miming. In other words, do not hinder the other areas—neither let them hinder you-- in your "high calling."

Of course, the exception is if you are multi-talented and can perform in more than one area, you shouldn't be hindered from doing so. However, if excellence is your goal, you will have to decide to advance one, or at most two, areas to increase your ministry effectiveness.

2) Do not despise the gifts of the other areas of Christian Dance. That is not just within your particular dance troupe, but in the dance area of the Body of Christ at large. You may not have a theatrical dance team/department who excels in technique, but you should not despise such teams or refer to their ministry as "un-anointed." Likewise, those senior ladies who can only wave a flag are just as anointed as you who minister choreographies for special presentations.

3) Contribute but do not control. Each area can use objective input from the others, but be sure that you provide yours in the spirit of edification, not arrogance or control.

4) Teach each other occasionally. Attend a workshop presented by, or conduct one for, the other areas. Whether it be mime, technique, theatre, prophetic, worship, or choreography, you'll be surprised at how much creativity this may inject into your particular ministry area.

Final Thoughts

Well, I hope that this text has brought you several steps closer to your enlarged territory in Christian Dance. Thank you so much for reading this resource and I hope that you will desire to further your studies with us by purchasing all the books in this series. In fact, you might want to take this time to review the Additional Resources section at back, which contains a list of our multimedia resources - i.e. textbooks, children's books, technique manuals, music cds, videos and e-Seminars–all under the **Dominion Dancer Series** label.

Also, for those who have not yet proceeded onto the online **VIRTUE Seminar Certificate (VSC) - or e-Seminar - program**, I must tell you that you are really missing out on a lot more than what we can present in this mere text form. Our

interactive Online Campus presents tools and resources that will take you much closer to experiencing your "enlarged territory," plus earn you a
3-credit Certificate upon completion. Please go
to www.DominionDancer.com for further information, as well as up-to-the-minute news updates
from our **blog**.

Once there, I urge you to register for *FREE
membership* in our **Dominion Dancer Network
(DDN)**, so that you can: (a) be among the first
to learn about the release dates for our books,
videos, and other multi-media resources; (b) take
advantage of membership discounts on selected
resources *(10-25%)*, seasonal coupons and special
privileges; (c) interact in real time with dancers
from around the world; and (d) view and submit
your own articles, discussion posts, live chat con-
versations, plus classified ads re: your upcoming
events, items for sale and professional services, all
for FREE!

Additionally, you can learn more about
upgrading your professional and academic
credentials via our very fulfilling **Degree and
Teaching Certification programs–featuring AA,**

BA, MA and PhD in Christian Dance Theatre. Please see details on our Certification page at www.dominionDancer.com. If you need any further information please **contact me directly** at any of the following:

> *Phone:* **242-380-8027;**
> *Fax:* **242-394-8383;**
> *Postal Address:*
> **Palmdale, PO Box SB-51351,**
> **Nassau, Bahamas;**
> *Email* **dominion_dancer@yahoo.com.**

Kingdom Dancer, like Abraham our father of faith, I pray that you be blessed perpetually and be a perpetual blessing!

> Forever In His Service,
> Professor M. T. Deveaux

End Notes

The author credits the teachings of Dr. Turnel Nelson and Dr. Myles Munroe, plus Chapter 12 of the book, *What If Jesus Had Never Been Born?* by Dr. D. James Kennedy and Jerry Newcombe, for influencing some of the viewpoints expressed herein.

Additional Resources
Edu-mercial

The Dominion Dancer Series–Multi-Media Resources List
www.DominionDancer.com
Continue Your Journey With These Diverse Resources!

1) Dominion Dancer TEXTBOOK Series

Exercising Kingdom Dominion In Dance

Dominion Strategies For Dance *Education*

Dominion Strategies For Dance *Artistry*

Dominion Strategies For Dance *Ministry*

Dominion Strategies For Dance *Business Administration*

2) Dominion Dancer CHILDREN'S BOOK Series

For kinder-dancers (Age 3 to 5 years)

For elementary dancers (Age 6 to 8 years)

For junior dancers (Age 9 to 12 years)

3) Dominion Dancer TECHNIQUE MANUAL Series

(Abbreviation: VCC = VIRTUE Completion Certificate).

Manual/Stage 1A–Part 1: VCC Levels K3, K4, & 1

Manual/Stage 1A–Part 2: VCC Levels 2 & 3

Manual/Stage 1B: VCC Level 4

Manual/Stage 1C: VCC Level 5

Manual/Stage 2A: VCC Level 6

Manual/Stage 2B: VCC Level 7

Manual/Stage 2C: VCC Level 8

Manual/Stage 3A: VCC Level 9

Manual/Stage 3B: VCC Level 10

Manual/Stage 3C: VCC Level 11

Manual/Stage 4: VCC Level 12

4) Dominion Dancer MUSIC CD Series

CD-1: Stage 1

CD-2: Stage 2

CD-3: Stage 3

CD-4: Stage 4

5) Dominion Dancer VIDEO Series

Video/Stage 1A–Part 1: VCC Levels K3, K4, & 1

Video/Stage 1A–Part 2: VCC Levels 2 & 3

Video/Stage 1B: VCC Level 4

Video/Stage 1C: VCC Level 5

Video/Stage 2A: VCC Level 6

Video/Stage 2B: VCC Level 7

Video/Stage 2C: VCC Level 8

Video/Stage 3A: VCC Level 9

Video/Stage 3B: VCC Level 10

Video/Stage 3C: VCC Level 11

Video/Stage 4: VCC Level 12

6) Dominion Dancer E-SEMINAR Series

(Below is the list of online courses, aka e-Seminars, their subject code numbers, seminar topics and program subject titles. The code abbreviations are represented as follows: MIN = Ministry, BUS = Business, EDU = Education, ART = Artistic).

MIN-111: *"Excercising Kingdom Dominion In Dance"*
> **Professional Development**

BUS-111: *"Establishing A Web-presence"*
> **Intro To Electronic Media**

EDU-111: *"VCC Exercises, Level K3, K4 & 1"*
> **Ballet Technique 1**

MIN-121: *"Prior Learning Achievement"*
> **Ministry Development 1**

BUS-121: *"Net Profit Resulsts"*
> **Electronic Media Development**

MIN-132: *"Dance Ministry Checklist, Struggles & Triumphs"*
> **Dance Theology**

MIN-242: *"Continued Learning Achievement"*
> **Ministry Development 2**

MIN-253: *"The History Of Dance In The Church"*
> **Dance History & Development**

EDU-121: *"VCC Exercises, Levels 2 & 3"*
> **Ballet Technique 2**

EDU-132: *"Lesson Planning & Execution, VCC Levels K3 & K4"*
Teaching Practice 1

EDU-242: *"Lesson Planning & Execution, VCC Level 1"*
Teaching Practice 2

EDU-253: *"Exam Preparation, VCC Levels K3, K4 & 1"*
Teaching Practice 3

ART-111: *"The Art Of Theatre"*
Dance Theatre Theory 1

ART-121: *"Recipe For A Successful Theatrical Production"*
Dance Theatre Theory 2

BUS-132: *"Principles Of Business Administration"*
Business Administration Principles

ART -132: *"Comparative Analysis Of Christian Versus Secular Show"*
Dance Appreciation

BUS-242: *"Dance Entity Administration, Principles & Practice"*
Business Administration Practice

ART-242: *"Movement Principles & Applications"*
Dance Technique Theory

BUS-253: *"Accounting With Quickbooks"*
Computerized Accounting

ART-253: *"Constructing An Original Theatrical Dance Show"*
Dance Theatre Practice 1

ART-263: *"Debut Of An Original Theatrical Dance Show"*
Dance Theatre Practice 2

BUS-263: *"Event Planning, Execution & Review"*
    Event Planning Strategies
MIN-263: *"Researching & Presenting A Dance Seminar"*
    Research & Speech Communication
EDU-263: *"Exam Concert, VCC Levels K3, K4 & 1"*
    Exam Theatre 1

For full details on each of these listings, along with up-to-the-minute news updates from our blog, plus details about joining our Dominion Dancer Network (DDN) or enrolling in our Degree & Teaching Certification programs, please visit us at: www.DominionDancer.com

Contact Marilyn Deveaux at
dominion_dancer@yahoo.com
or order more copies of this book at

Tate Publishing, LLC

127 East Trade Center Terrace
Mustang, Oklahoma 73064

(888) 361 - 9473

Tate Publishing, Llc
www.tatepublishing.com